Pregnancy-friendly meal plan:

A week-by-week pregnancy meal plan and nutrition guide to ensure that you and your unborn child eat healthily throughout your pregnancy

By
Darla B. Humphrey

Copyright :

Disclaimer:

The data given in this. [Pregnancy-friendly meal plan] is for general enlightening purposes as it were. It isn't expected to fill in for proficient clinical, legal, or monetary counsel. Perusers are urged to talk with proper experts for exhortations customised to their singular conditions.

The writer and distributor make no representations or guarantees with respect to the precision, fulfilment, or reasonableness of the data contained.

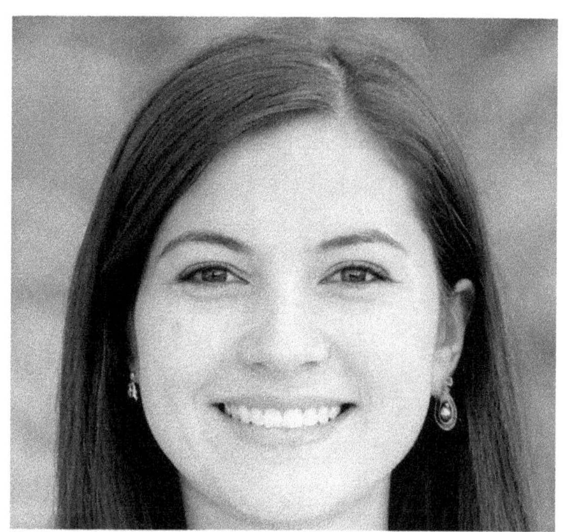

About the author

Dala B. Humphrey remains a signal of skill and empathy in the domain of maternal consideration and pre-birth nourishment. A recognized medical caretaker and expert in the field, she has committed her profession to improving the prosperity of eager moms and advancing the sound improvement of unborn youngsters.

With a rich foundation in nursing, Humphrey brings a remarkable mix of clinical information and compassionate comprehension to her work. Her energy for supporting ladies through the groundbreaking excursion of pregnancy drove her to spend significant time on pre-birth sustenance, perceiving the significant effect that eating regimen and sustenance have on the wellbeing and imperativeness of both mother and youngster.

Humphrey's obligation to confirm-based rehearsals is obvious in her careful way to deal with creating the pregnancy-friendly meal plan. Her skill goes beyond the clinical, reaching out into a domain where sustenance turns into a foundation for cultivating profound prosperity and association during the pre-birth venture.

Notwithstanding her expert honours, Humphrey's glow and compassion radiate through her associations with hopeful moms. She grasps the extraordinary difficulties and delights that pregnancy brings, and her direction isn't just established in clinical skill but additionally in a profound appreciation for the close-to-home and groundbreaking nature of parenthood.

As a writer, Humphrey welcomes perusers into a reality where each page is a demonstration of her commitment to engaging ladies with information and backing. The pregnancy-friendly meal plan isn't simply an impression of her mastery, but a sign of her confidence in the all-encompassing way to deal with maternal consideration, where sustaining the body is entwined with supporting the soul.

Dala B. Humphrey's commitments stretch out past the composed word; she remains a consoling presence for those exploring the mind-boggling scene of pregnancy. Her work is an encouragement to set out on an excursion of taking care of oneself, shrewdness, and festivity, directed by a sympathetic master who comprehends that the magnificence of pregnancy lies in the fragile equilibrium of actual wellbeing, close-to-home prosperity, and the delight of carrying new life into the world.

Bonus

Pregnancy: what to eat and what to avoid

Introduction

Dala B. Humphrey stays as a sign of expertise and compassion in the space of maternal thought and pre-birth sustenance. A perceived clinical overseer and master in the field, she has committed her calling to working on the thriving of enthusiastic mothers and propelling the sound improvement of unborn young people.

With a rich background in nursing, Humphrey brings a wonderful blend of clinical data and empathetic perception to her work. Her energy for supporting women through the noteworthy journey of pregnancy drove her to invest critical time in pre-birth food, seeing the massive impact that eating routine and food have on the prosperity and essentialness of both mother and adolescent.

Humphrey's commitment to affirmative-based practices is clear in her cautious manner in making the pregnancy-friendly meal plan. Her expertise goes beyond the clinical, connecting into a space where food transforms into an establishment for developing significant flourishing and relationships during the pre-birth adventure.

Despite her master's praise, Humphrey's shine and sympathy emanate through her relationship with confident mothers. She gets a handle on the remarkable challenges and enjoyments that pregnancy brings, and her heading isn't simply settled in clinical expertise yet furthermore in a significant appreciation for the up-close, personal, and historic nature of being a parent.

As a writer, Humphrey invites perusers into a reality where each page is an exhibition of her obligation to draw in women with data and support. The pregnancy-friendly meal plan isn't just an impression of her dominance; it's an indication of her trust in a comprehensive manner to manage maternal thought, where supporting the body is laced with supporting the spirit.

Dala B. Humphrey's responsibilities loosen up past the created word; she stays as a supporting presence for those investigating the marvellous scene of pregnancy. Her work is a consolation to set out on a journey of dealing with oneself, cleverness, and celebration, coordinated by a thoughtful expert who fathoms that the grandness of pregnancy lies in the delicate harmony of genuine prosperity, near and dear success, and the pleasure of conveying new life into the world

Chapter 1

Overview of pregnancy nutrition

- ## Comprehending Nutrition in Pregnancy:

Prenatal nutrition, a crucial component of both maternal and fetal health, affects the mother's and the developing child's health throughout the pregnancy.

This thorough methodology includes tending to different aspects, including the meaning of nourishment during pregnancy, normal healthful worries, and exposing legends related to pregnancy counts and calories.

• The Value of Eating Well During Pregnancy:

Increased nutritional needs during pregnancy in order to support the mother's body's physiological changes and to encourage the best possible development of the fetus.

Key supplements, for example, folic corrosive, iron, calcium, and omega-3 unsaturated fats, assume vital roles in forestalling birth deserts, guaranteeing legitimate organ arrangement, and supporting the development of the hatchling.

Nourishment during pregnancy isn't just about the amount of food; it's also about the quality. A balanced eating routine that incorporates various natural products, such as vegetables, whole grains, lean proteins, and dairy items, gives the fundamental nutrients and minerals necessary for a solid pregnancy. Insufficient sustenance during this basic period can prompt complexities, for example, preterm birth, low birth weight, and formative issues.

- **Typical nutritional issues:**

Pregnancy-related nutritional concerns are caused by a number of factors. If the body's increased need for certain nutrients, altered metabolism, and increased energy requirements are not properly addressed, deficiencies may result. For example, iron deficiency can cause anaemia, which puts the mother and the unborn child at risk.

Furthermore, conditions like preeclampsia and gestational diabetes emphasize how crucial it is to control blood sugar levels and eat a balanced diet. Handling common issues requires customized diet advice, consistent observation, and supplementation as needed. Pregnant women need guidance from healthcare providers to navigate these nutritional challenges.

• **Dispelling Untruths Regarding Pregnancy Diets:**

Expectant mothers are often confused by the plethora of advice and myths surrounding the dietary choices that accompany pregnancy. Clarifying the myths surrounding the designation of certain foods as "off-limits" and severe dietary restrictions is crucial. For example, while avoiding unpasteurized products and raw fish is a good precaution, eliminating a particular food group entirely can result in nutritional imbalances.

Women are better equipped to make decisions when they are informed about the benefits of a varied diet, the necessity of extra calories, and the safety of moderate caffeine consumption. Dispelling myths guarantees that expectant people receive accurate

Chapter 2

Summary of the pregnancy's three trimesters:

First trimester:

The first trimester lasts from week 1 to week 12 and is very important for the development of an undeveloped organism. During this period, the processed eggs develop into tiny humans with improved major organs and structures. As hormones change, mothers may experience fatigue, emotional outbursts, and morning sickness. During this semester, prenatal care will be accelerated, with regular check-ups to monitor the health of the mother and the child's development.

Second Trimester:

The second trimester, which usually lasts from the 13th week to the 26th week of pregnancy, is considered to be the most comfortable period of pregnancy. As for the underlying problem, some symptoms, such as morning sickness, for example, usually disappear, and the mother usually experiences an increase in energy. The fetus develops rapidly during this pregnancy, and the child's organs are still developing. The mother may begin to sense the development of the fetus, and a normal ultrasound filter can detect the orientation of the fetus.

Third trimester of pregnancy:

The final stage, lasting from week 27 to week 40, includes the completion of the fetal transition and the building of the basis for delivery. As the uterus grows, the mother becomes more anxious and more aware of her child's growth. Prenatal visits to measure the mother's pulse, assess the child's condition, and evaluate the general health of both parties are becoming increasingly common. Additionally, there are high expectations for your work and performance this semester. Expectant parents often take birth preparation classes, plan for a home birth, and plan daycare in preparation for the impending birth. Toward the end of the third trimester, your child may be in a head-down position. This indicates that they are ready to give birth.

Each trimester appears to have unique needs throughout the pregnancy, from laying the foundation for life in the first trimester to promoting strong development in the second trimester to preparing for the miraculous event of childbirth in the third trimester. I'm satisfied. Being close to home and experiencing real change over the last few weeks adds to the wonderful experience of taking on a guardianship role.

Chapter 3

Incorporating Essential Nutrients

- **Folate**

Also known as synthetic folic acid, it is a B vitamin that is extremely important, especially during pregnancy. Let's explore its importance and how it affects the health of the mother and fetus.

The importance of folic acid during pregnancy:

1. Neural tube development: Folic acid helps prevent spina bifida. It plays an important

role in preventing neural tube defects such as anencephaly and anencephaly. in the first weeks of pregnancy. Therefore, it is especially important to ensure sufficient folic acid intake before pregnancy and during the early stages of pregnancy.

2: Red blood cell production: Folic acid is required for the production of red blood cells, which are important for transporting oxygen throughout the body.

Sources of folate:

1. Food Sources: Good sources of folate include dark leafy vegetables (spinach, kale), lentils, beans, citrus fruits, avocados, and fortified grain products.
2. Dietary supplements: Many prenatal vitamins contain folic acid, which can help pregnant women meet their daily folic acid needs.

Recommended intake:

The recommended intake of folic acid for pregnant women is 600 micrograms per day. It is worth noting that because the formation of the neural tube occurs very early in pregnancy, often before a woman even realizes she is pregnant, it is recommended that women of childbearing age consume sufficient folic acid before becoming pregnant. Worth it. Risk of folate deficiency: Insufficient folic acid intake during pregnancy can increase the risk of neural tube defects and cause anemia in the mother.

Tips to ensure adequate folate intake:

1. Nutritious diet: Eat a variety of foods rich in folate, including leafy greens, legumes, and fortified grains.
2. Pregnancy Supplements: To bridge the gap and ensure adequate folic acid intake, consider taking a pregnancy vitamin that contains folic acid. It is usually

recommended that you start taking prenatal vitamins before you become pregnant.

Nutritional fortification and public health initiatives:

Many countries have implemented fortification programs by adding folic acid to certain foods, such as grains and cereals, to ensure that individuals, especially pregnant women, meet their folic acid needs. I am.

Consultation with your healthcare provider:

It is important to discuss your specific dietary and nutritional needs with your health care provider, as they can provide you with personalized advice about folic acid intake and supplements during pregnancy.

Ensuring optimal folic acid intake is an important part of prenatal care and lays the foundation for the healthy development of the baby and the well-being of the mother during pregnancy.

- **Iron**

It is an essential nutrient during pregnancy, supporting both the mother's health and the baby's development. Let's take a closer look at the importance of iron during pregnancy and how it affects the health of the mother and fetus.

- The importance of iron during pregnancy:
1. Oxygen Transport: Iron is an important component of oxygen. Hemoglobin is a protein within red blood cells. Transports oxygen to cells and tissues. During pregnancy, the mother's blood volume increases to support the growth of the fetus. Therefore, an adequate supply of iron is required to produce these additional red blood cells.

2: Fetal Development: Iron is essential for the development of your baby's own red blood cell supply and overall growth.

- Iron Sources:
1. Food Sources: Good sources of iron include lean red meat, poultry, fish, lentils, beans, tofu, fortified grains, and dark leafy greens such as spinach and kale. Contains vegetables.
2. Dietary supplements: Many prenatal vitamins contain iron and can help pregnant women meet their daily iron needs.

- Recommended Intake:

The recommended daily intake of iron for pregnant women is 27 milligrams, which is significantly higher than the recommended intake for non-pregnant women. This increase is necessary to increase blood volume and support the baby's need for red blood cell production.

- Risk of iron deficiency:

Insufficient iron intake during pregnancy can lead to iron deficiency anemia in the mother, causing fatigue and weakness and leading to premature birth and a low birth weight for the baby. may cause an increased risk of

- Tips for ensuring adequate iron intake:
1. Eating iron-rich foods: heme iron (found in animal foods) and non-heme iron

(found in animal foods) Include a variety of iron-rich foods in your diet, including both. (Contains herbal products.).

2. Prenatal supplements: If your dietary iron intake is inadequate, consider taking a prenatal vitamin containing iron to ensure you meet your daily needs.

- Considerations and Advice:

As with other nutrients, it is important to discuss your specific nutritional and dietary needs with your doctor to ensure that your individual iron needs are met during pregnancy. Your health care provider can give you personalized advice and monitor your iron levels through blood tests.

Adequate iron intake is an important part of prenatal care as it supports the overall health and well-being of both the mother and the developing baby.

- Calcium

Calcium plays a significant role in pregnancy, supporting the general wellbeing and improvement of both the mother and her developing child. We should investigate the significance of calcium during pregnancy and its different impacts:

- The significance of calcium during pregnancy:
1. Bone turn of events: Calcium is essential for heart development and helps your baby's bones, teeth, and muscles. The child gets the calcium it needs from the mother's stores, so it is critical that the

mother keep up with sufficient calcium levels.

2: Maternal wellbeing: Calcium upholds the mother's bone wellbeing by assisting the mother with keeping up with her own bone thickness.

Calcium Sources:

1. Food Sources: Great wellsprings of calcium incorporate dairy items like milk, cheddar, and yogurt, plant-strengthened milks (for example, almond milk and soy milk), green verdant vegetables (for example, kale), calcium-braced food varieties like kale, juices, and cereals.
2. Dietary Enhancements: Pre-birth nutrients frequently contain calcium, if necessary, to assist pregnant ladies with meeting their day-to-day calcium needs.

Suggested consumption:

For women between the ages of 19 and 50, the daily allowance of calcium for pregnant women is 1,000 milligrams. During the last two trimesters of pregnancy, the child's bones grow quickly, so the requirement for calcium increases.

- Calcium Deficiency Danger:

Lacking calcium admission during pregnancy implies that the child gets the calcium it needs straightforwardly from the mother's bones, which can debilitate the mother's bone thickness. Additionally, it may have an impact on your baby's bone development.

- Ways to get legitimate calcium consumption:
1. Eating calcium-rich food sources: Remember calcium-rich food varieties for your eating routine and attempt to join dairy and plant sources to guarantee assortment and equilibrium.

2. Pre-birth supplements: On the off chance that dietary calcium intake is inadequate, consider taking a pre-birth nutrient containing calcium to meet everyday necessities.

- Conference with your medical care supplier:

To make sure you get the calcium you need when you're pregnant, it's important to talk to your doctor about your specific dietary and nutritional requirements. We will give individualized guidance and suggest calcium supplementation if it is fundamental.

Guaranteeing sufficient calcium admission upholds the sound advancement of your child's bones and keeps up with your own bone wellbeing during pregnancy and beyond.

- **Omega-3 fatty acids**

assumes a critical role in supporting the wellbeing and improvement of both the mother and the developing child during pregnancy. We should investigate the significance of omega-3 unsaturated fats during this basic period.

- The Significance of Omega-3 Unsaturated Fats During Pregnancy:
1. Development of the Fetal Brain and Eye: Omega-3 unsaturated fats, especially DHA (docosahexaenoic corrosive), are fundamental for the advancement of the child's mind and eyes.
2. Maternal Wellbeing: Omega-3 unsaturated fats offer advantages for the mother's cardiovascular and general wellbeing during this time of expanding metabolic demands.

- Wellsprings of Omega-3 Unsaturated Fats:

1. Greasy Fish: Fatty fish like salmon, mackerel, trout, and sardines are excellent sources of omega-3 fatty acids. Additionally, these fish are low in mercury, making them a safe option for pregnant women.

2. Plant-Based Sources: Omega-3 fatty acids can be obtained from plant-based sources like flaxseeds, chia seeds, and walnuts for individuals who do not consume fish.

3. Supplementation: Pregnant women may likewise think about omega-3 enhancements, especially those containing DHA, to guarantee satisfactory admission.

- Suggested Admission:

The suggested intake of omega-3 unsaturated fats during pregnancy incorporates somewhere around 200–300 milligrams of DHA each day. The baby's development of the brain and eyes is aided by this intake.

- Dangers of Omega-3 Inadequacy:

Omega-3 fatty acid deficiency during pregnancy may have an effect on the neurological development of the unborn child, potentially affecting cognitive function, visual acuity, and overall brain health.

- Contemplations and Meetings:

It's vital to examine your particular dietary and nourishing necessities with a medical care supplier to guarantee that you are meeting your singular omega-3 unsaturated fat prerequisites during pregnancy. They can offer individual guidance and, if necessary, may suggest omega-3 supplements.

By guaranteeing sufficient omega-3 unsaturated fat admission, you're supporting the sound improvement of the child's cerebrum and eyes while additionally advancing your own cardiovascular and by-and-large wellbeing during pregnancy.

- **Protein**

is a fundamental supplement during pregnancy, supporting the development and improvement of the child and assisting with keeping up with the mother's general wellbeing. We should plunge into the significance of protein during pregnancy and its different effects:

Significance of Protein During Pregnancy:

1. Growth and Development of the Fetus: Protein is a key structural block for the development and improvement of the child, supporting the arrangement of organs, muscles, and tissues.
2. Health for Mothers: Protein is critical for the support and fixation of the mother's own tissues, including muscle, skin, and platelets.

Wellsprings of Protein:

1. Creature-Based Sources: Lean meats, poultry, fish, eggs, and dairy items are rich wellsprings of superior-grade, complete protein.
2. Plant-Based Sources: Plant-based protein can be obtained from nuts, seeds, tofu, quinoa, beans, lentils, and other legumes.

Suggested Admission:

The suggested daily intake of protein for pregnant women is around 71 grams. This expanded requirement for protein means a lot for the fast development and improvement of the child.

Dangers of a Lack of Protein:

Insufficient protein admission during pregnancy can influence the child's development and improvement, possibly prompting low birth weight and other formative issues. For the mother, a lack of protein intake might influence her general wellbeing and recuperation during and after pregnancy.

Ways to Guarantee Sufficient Protein Admission:

1. Adjusted Diet: Consume a blend of excellent creature-based and plant-based

protein sources to guarantee assortment and equilibrium in your eating routine.

2. Supplementation: Assuming that dietary admission is deficient, medical care suppliers might propose protein supplementation, particularly when cravings are impacted by pregnancy-related side effects.

Conference with Medical Services Suppliers:

Examining explicit dietary and wholesome necessities with a medical services supplier is vital to guaranteeing that you are meeting your singular protein prerequisites during pregnancy. They may address any concerns regarding protein intake and offer individualized guidance.

By guaranteeing satisfactory protein admission, you're supporting the sound development and improvement of the child while likewise keeping up with your own wellbeing and prosperity all through pregnancy and then some

- **Iodine**

is a critical mineral during pregnancy, assuming an imperative role in supporting the prosperity of both the mother and the child. Here is a more critical glance at iodine and its importance during pregnancy:

Significance of iodine during pregnancy:

1. Thyroid Capability: Thyroid hormones contain iodine, which is a necessary component that controls important physiological processes like metabolism

and brain and nervous system development.

2. Growth of the Fetus: Satisfactory iodine admission is especially basic during pregnancy, as it straightforwardly influences the child's mental health and, generally speaking, development. Lacking iodine can prompt hindered development and scholarly handicaps in the child.

3. Maternal Wellbeing: Iodine additionally upholds the mother's thyroid capability during the expanded metabolic demands of pregnancy.

Wellsprings of Iodine:

1. Diet: Iodine can be gotten from different dietary sources, including iodized salt, dairy items, fish (with some restraint), ocean growth, and some business bread.

2. Supplements: Pre-birth nutrients frequently contain iodine to assist with

guaranteeing that pregnant people meet their everyday necessities.

Suggested Admission:

The suggested day-to-day admission of iodine during pregnancy is 220 micrograms. This is somewhat higher than the general suggested admission for non-pregnant adults, as the interest in iodine increments during pregnancy helps the child's neurological turn of events.

Threats from iodine deficiency:

Lacking iodine utilization during pregnancy can incite a range of troublesome outcomes, including:

Maternal hypothyroidism: This can provoke complexities like pre-eclampsia, preterm birth, and fruitless work.

Damage to the fetus's brain: the iodine need of the mother can cause irreversible neurological mischief in the youngster, influencing mental development and potentially provoking cretinism.

Step-by step instructions to ensure you get sufficient iodine:

1. Eat food sources high in iodine.
   Coordinate iodine-rich food sources into your eating routine, such as iodized salt, dairy products, and fish. In any case, due to the potential mercury content, it is essential to consume fish with caution.
2. Supplements for Pregnancy: If your dietary confirmation of iodine is missing, consider using pre-birth supplements that integrate iodine to help with breaking any boundaries.

To no one's surprise, it's basic to inspect your specific dietary and supporting necessities with a clinical benefits provider to ensure that you are meeting your particular iodine essentials during pregnancy.

Chapter 4

Beyond Nutrition: Emotional Well-being During Pregnancy

Emotional Well-being Pregnancy is a fundamentally significant part of prenatal care, impacting both the mother's and the child's wellbeing. How about we investigate a few critical contemplations and methodologies to help profound health during this time?

The Significance of Emotional Well-Being During Pregnancy

1. Influence on Maternal Wellbeing: Close to Home Emotion can influence the mother's general wellbeing and may impact

pregnancy-related side effects like sickness, exhaustion, and stress.

2. Consequences for the Fetal Turn of Events: The mother's personal state can affect the child's turn of events and possibly impact their drawn-out prosperity.

Key Contemplations:

1. StressThe executives: Overseeing pressure through unwinding methods, care, and looking for daily encouragement can emphatically affect maternal wellbeing and the fetal turn of events.

2. Open Correspondence: Open communication with a network of people who can support you, like your doctor, partner, family, and friends, can help you deal with your emotional issues and feel more at ease.

3. **Self-Care:** Focusing on taking care of oneself through exercises like delicate activity, agreeable side interests, and sufficient rest can uphold close-to-home prosperity.
4. **Readiness and Instruction:** Finding out about pregnancy, labor, and postpartum care can mitigate nervousness and lift trust in the excursion ahead.

Decreasing Tension and Sorrow:

1. **Professional Assistance:** It is essential to seek professional emotional health support, such as counselling or therapy, in the event of anxiety or depression.
2. **Treatments supervised by doctors:** Medical care suppliers can give direction on the safe and powerful administration of tension or sorrow during pregnancy, including drugs when vital.

Accomplices and Social Help:

1. **Accomplice Inclusion:** Empowering accomplices to take part in the pregnancy cycle can be a priceless wellspring of consistent encouragement for the eager mother.
2. **Social Association:** Keeping up with social associations with loved ones, as well as searching out help gatherings, can give a feeling of local area and understanding during this time.

Care and unwinding:

1. **Care Practices:** Care-based exercises like reflection, profound breathing activities, and pre-birth yoga can assist with overseeing pressure and advance close-to-home prosperity.
2. **Positive Confirmations:** Participating in sure self-talk and confirmations can assist

with developing a feeling of quiet and certainty.

Medical Services Supplier Joint effort:

Transparent correspondence with medical services suppliers is vital, empowering them to give customized direction and backing in view of the person's close-to-home prosperity needs during pregnancy.

By focusing on profound prosperity, hopeful moms can decidedly affect their own wellbeing and the general insight of pregnancy. Searching out help, keeping up with solid survival methods, and encouraging positive close-to-home associations can contribute to a more certain and satisfying pregnancy venture.

In the event that you have explicit inquiries regarding close-to-home prosperity during pregnancy or require further direction on related subjects, go ahead and inquire!

Chapter 5

Crafting a Pregnancy-Friendly Meal Plan

Building balanced meals:

Focusing on creating balanced meals that provide different supplements necessary for the mother and the developing child is crucial during pregnancy. Don't withhold anything from solid fats, proteins, carbohydrates, or a variety of vitamins and minerals. To ensure a well-rounded nutritional profile, include whole grains, lean proteins, natural products, vegetables, and dairy or dairy alternatives. Maintaining portion control is essential to preventing excessive weight gain while still fulfilling the increased nutritional needs during pregnancy.

A plan for a pregnancy meal:

A pregnancy meal plan is a tool for organizing wholesome, well-balanced dinners to support the health of the expectant mother and her unborn child. It typically recalls a variety of food types high in essential nutrients such as protein, calcium, iron, folate, and omega-3 unsaturated fats. Lean proteins, vegetables, whole grains, natural products, and dairy or dairy alternatives could all be included in a well-balanced pregnancy dinner plan.

An example of a pregnancy dinner plan would look something like this:

- Leafy foods are rich in fibre, minerals, and nutrients.

- Whole grains are excellent sources of energy and essential nutrients.

- Lean meats, chicken, fish, beans, lentils, and tofu are good sources of protein.

- Dairy or Choices: foods high in calcium, such as yogurt, milk, and other sustained plant-based alternatives.

- Solid Fats: The main sources of unsaturated fats are avocado, nuts, seeds, and olive oil.

- Iron-Dense Food Types: Lean meats, beans, spinach, and braced grains are good sources of iron.

- Vegetables, organic citrus products, and salad greens are good sources of folate for fetal development.

It is imperative that expectant mothers discuss their specific dietary needs, illnesses, and dietary restrictions with their medical services provider or a registered dietitian in order to personalize the meal plan.

A detailed meal plan for pregnant women:

Although specific nutritional needs vary, this is a general weekly pregnancy meal plan. Adjust segment sizes based on your own needs.

- Weeks 1 through 12: Emphasize whole grains, vegetables, lean proteins, and organic goods.

Drink plenty of water to stay hydrated.

Keep in mind foods like spinach, lentils, and citrus-based natural products that are high in iron and folate.

- Weeks 13–28: Increase calcium intake in conjunction with dairy or other braced plant-based options to help children's bones grow. For mental health, omega-3 unsaturated fats are essential; try including pecans, chia seeds, and salmon.

- Weeks 29–36: Add extra protein to your child's diet by including eggs, vegetables, and poultry.

Consume foods high in iron, such as salad greens and lean red meat, to prevent pallor.

- Weeks 37–40: Increase your intake of foods like complex carbohydrates and protein that will give you more energy and stamina while working.

For mental well-being, stay hydrated and include sources of solid fats.

Consult a nutritionist or your healthcare provider for personalized advice based on your unique needs for well-being during pregnancy.

Overall Advice:

- Frequent Mini-Feasts: Eating smaller, more frequent dinners helps control diabetes and prevent illness.

- Bright Plate: A variety of lovely soil products ensures a range of supplements. Nothing should be left on your plate.
- Minimize the variety of handled food: Reduce your intake of processed and high-sugar foods; instead, focus on adding healthy options to your diet for your overall well-being.
- Speak with a Medical Provider: Regularly consult with a medical professional qualified to customize the meal plan to each person's needs and take care of a specific health issue.

Chapter 6

Exercise and Real Work:

Maintaining a regular exercise regimen every day while pregnant is essential for the health of the mother and the unborn child. Low-impact activities that promote a steady weight gain, lessen discomfort, and enhance dissemination include swimming, walking, and prenatal yoga. However, it's essential to consult a medical services professional before starting any exercise program to make sure it aligns with the individual's health status and the specific requirements of the pregnancy.

Guidelines for Prenatal Exercise:

- Focus on moderate-intensity workouts.

- Steer clear of high-influence activities that could be risky.

- Include pelvic floor exercises to improve your muscle strength.

- Observe Your Body: Pay attention to how your body reacts and functions.

- Adapt your exercise routine to the circumstances and avoid overdoing it.

- Drink plenty of water and take breaks when necessary.

Benefits of Exercise During Pregnancy:

improved disposition and less stress.

Reduced back pain and improved performance.

increased vitality and improved quality of sleep.

Relaxing and resting:

Getting enough sleep is essential for a healthy pregnancy. Unsettling influences on sleep are common, especially as a pregnancy progresses, but excellent sleep hygiene practices can completely improve sleep.

Make a loosening-up plan. Schedule for sleep:

Before going to bed, create a peaceful environment.

Avoid animating exercises right before bedtime.

Consider doing some delicate extending or prenatal yoga.

Optimal Resting Places:

Sleeping on the left side improves blood flow to the kidneys and uterus.

Use cushions for support and comfort.

Attending to Distresses at Rest:

Monitor nausea, leg cramps, and dyspepsia accompanying changes in lifestyle.

If necessary, speak with a medical services provider about safe tranquilizers. Support and Inclusion of Accomplices: Having a significant and practical accomplice is crucial during pregnancy. Encouraging dynamic inclusion fosters a sense of belonging and shared responsibility.

Direct communication with the partner

Analyze plans, assumptions, and worries in a clear and open manner.

- Attend pre-birth classes together to enhance comprehension.

Consistent motivation:

- Be considerate of your pregnant partner's emotions.
- Express feelings and participate in conversations about the pregnancy in an effective manner.
- Valuable Assistance: Assisting with household duties and planning for the child.
- Attend birthing classes and clinical arrangements together.

Keeping important doors open: Engage in activities that promote holding with the child, such as reading.

Chapter 7

Troubleshooting Common Challenges

Food aversion and nausea can be normal issues in various circumstances, including pregnancy, disease, and a few operations. To treat queasiness, it's vital to perceive the reason and keep away from it. Keeping up with your liquid intake and eating small, continuous meals might be beneficial. You can include peppermint and ginger in your diet, as they are known to have anti-nausea effects. Changing the consistency or temperature of what you eat can also help reduce

Cravings

Numerous things can cause cravings, like hormonal changes, dietary inadequacies, or close-to-home triggers. Stopping cravings can be supported by a nutritious eating routine. Eating a variety of food varieties and booking ordinary dinners helps keep blood sugar levels stable, which decreases the opportunity for serious desires. Successfully hankering the executives can be accomplished by perceiving close-to-home triggers and distinguishing substitute survival techniques, like practicing or rehearsing care.

Handling Aversions and Cravings

Recognizing Cravings: Recognize your cravings, but concentrate on choosing healthier options. For example, if you're craving something sweet, go for fruits or yogurt flavoured with honey rather than processed sugar.

Handling Aversions: If a particular food causes an aversion, look for appropriate substitutes that offer comparable nutrients. For instance, look into plant-based protein sources like beans if you can't handle meat. Investigate plant-based protein sources such as tofu or beans.

Drink enough water. This is especially important if you have a problem drinking plain water. Drink herbal teas or infuse water with fruits, but stay away from too much caffeine.

Taking Care of Nutritional Issues

Inadequate intake, dietary requirements, or imbalances can give rise to nutritional issues. It is imperative to adopt a diverse and well-rounded diet that includes essential nutrients in order to address these issues. A registered dietitian or nutritionist can offer tailored advice based on specific requirements and medical conditions. Using food journals or apps to track nutrient intake can help detect possible deficiencies. To develop a customized nutritional plan for individuals with particular dietary requirements or medical conditions, working with healthcare professionals is crucial. Frequent examinations and dietary modifications can guarantee continued nutritional health and wellness.

Keep in mind that each case is unique and that these notes are only broad recommendations. For precise and customized advice based on unique circumstances, always seek the counsel of healthcare professionals.

Chapter 8

Celebrating Motherhood

Embracing the Joy of Pregnancy:

Commending parenthood starts with the significant experience of pregnancy, an extraordinary excursion that gives pleasure, expectation, and a profound association between a mother and her unborn child. Embracing this period includes recognizing the physical and close-to-home changes, appreciating the supernatural occurrence of life developing inside, and finding delight in the one-of-a-kind bond that it creates.

During pregnancy, a lady goes through different actual changes, from the unobtrusive vacillating of the principal kicks to the recognizable development of the child knock. These changes, however testing on occasion, represent the making of life and the strength that accompanies supporting a new being. Embracing the delight of pregnancy includes delighting in the magnificence of this cycle, cultivating a positive mentality, and valuing the strength and flexibility of the female body.

Past the actual angles, embracing the delight of pregnancy is tied in with supporting close-to-home prosperity. Interfacing with the unborn youngster through snapshots of reflection, talking, and, in any event, playing music encourages a novel mother-kid bond. Encircling oneself with a steady local area, whether it be family, companions, or medical care experts, can additionally upgrade the delight of this groundbreaking period.

Getting ready for the appearance of your child:

As the excursion through pregnancy unfurls, the expectation and energy work towards the approaching appearance of the child. Getting ready for this huge occasion includes functional and profound perspectives, guaranteeing a smooth transition into parenthood.

From a down-to-earth perspective, moms participate in settling exercises, establishing an inviting climate for the infant. This includes setting up the nursery, putting together child basics, and making vital plans for the postpartum time frame. Teaching oneself about labor, newborn child care, and nurturing methods likewise assumes a pivotal role in planning for the appearance of the child.

Inwardly, planning for the child's appearance includes developing a sense of status and certainty. This might incorporate going to pre-birth classes, looking for counsel from experienced moms, and laying out an encouraging group of people. Embracing the obscure with a positive outlook and an open heart adds to smoother progress into the obligations of parenthood.

Bonus

Pregnancy: what to eat and what to avoid

Due to the risk of contracting Listeria monocytogenes, it has been announced that smoked fish, such as smoked salmon, should now be avoided if you are pregnant or otherwise considered vulnerable.

Smoked fish isn't the main food individuals who are pregnant ought to stay away from, and while attempting to figure out what's protected and what's viewed as high-risk, isolating reality from fiction can be confusing.

It's as much about including food sources that can be useful to your child for all intents and purposes as staying away from food sources that might be destructive. You shouldn't need to feel denied during these intriguing nine months, assuming that you know current realities.

Exhortation changes and varies from one country to another. This data is consistent with NHS counsel.

Foods to eat while you're pregnant:

With a few exceptions, pregnant women should eat the same healthy, varied diet that everyone else should. Eat a lot of products of the soil, wholegrains, lean meats, or vegan protein food sources like beans, lentils, and heartbeats. Hydrate, as well.

Pregnant ladies need to guarantee they are getting sufficient calcium, so attempt to incorporate lower-fat milk items like normal yogurt, semi-skimmed milk, or calcium-strengthened non-dairy items in your day-to-day diet.

Try not to be enticed to "eat for two." Pregnant ladies need shockingly few additional calories every day. You may reach for a quick pick-me-up in the confectionery aisle due to the inevitable fatigue and cravings. Choose slow-release energy foods that give you more of the vitamins and minerals you need instead of sweets and treats.

Food sources to check

- Fish and mercury

Shark, swordfish, and marlin are off the menu for pregnant ladies since they can contain enough mercury to hurt your child. Other, more modest slick fish can likewise contain mercury, so the guidance for pregnant ladies is to eat something like two 140-gram segments per seven-day stretch of mackerel, salmon, sardines, anchovies, trout, or other sleek fish.

All things considered, pregnant ladies ought to attempt to incorporate these two bits of slick fish to guarantee they get sufficient omega-3 unsaturated fats to help their developing child's mental health.

- Omega-3

Getting sufficient omega-3 during pregnancy is significant; however, it tends to be confusing to comprehend which food varieties give you what you really want.

Omega-3 unsaturated fats fall into two classifications:

ALA is found in a range of plant sources, including chia seeds, ground flaxseed, rapeseed oil, pecans, hazelnuts, walnuts, and green verdant vegetables. Since the body cannot produce ALA, it is essential to consume sufficient amounts from these sources. Omega-3-enhanced eggs are likewise a decent source.

DHA and EPA: long-chain omega-3 fats have significant advantages to mental health, particularly in pregnant ladies and small kids. The body can make these from ALA, but not as productively as consuming them straightforwardly. Fish oil and microalgae-based omega-3 enhancements are accessible, as are omega-3-improved eggs.

Fish liver oil enhancements ought to be kept away from in light of the fact that they likewise convey high levels of vitamin A.

- Cheddar

Delicate cheeses with a delicate white skin (brie, camembert, taleggio, and so forth) and delicate blue cheeses (gorgonzola, dolcelatte, and Danish blue) ought to be avoided, except if they are cooked until steaming hot the whole way through. This is on the grounds that they might convey listeria, which can cause a difficult ailment in pregnancy.

Hard cheeses, for example, Cheddar, Parmesan, and stilton, are fine to eat, regardless of whether they are made with unpasteurized milk. The high aridity and low water content of these cheeses make them unfriendly spots for microbes to develop.

Delicate cheeses produced using sanitized milk are okay to eat as well. Really take a look at the marks on mozzarella, feta, halloumi, ricotta, goat's cheese, and paneer.

- Eggs

The exhortation on half-cooked eggs in pregnancy changed in 2017. It's presently viewed as protected to eat crude or delicately cooked hen's eggs on the off chance that they convey the English Lion mark stepped on the shell. This imprint shows that the maker has stuck to the Lion Code of Training, and the eggs will be liberated from salmonella.

On the off chance that you have eggs from a neighbour or another source, make certain to cook both the white and yolk completely prior to eating.

Always cook the eggs of duck, goose, and quail thoroughly.

- Energized drinks

While having some caffeine is fine, the exhortation isn't to surpass 200 mg each day. Consumption of a lot of caffeine has been linked to low birthweight in infants. The amount of caffeine in coffee-based and flavoured drinks varies greatly. A medium cappuccino from a high-end chain could contain up to 195 mg of caffeine. By and large, a cup of tea contains 75mg of caffeine, and a cup of instant espresso contains 100mg of caffeine. A cup of channel or cafetiere espresso contains around 135 mg of caffeine.

On the off chance that you can't confront surrendering your espresso during pregnancy, change to decaf or even mix decaf and standard espresso to make a "

Food varieties to stay away from

* Smoked fish

Because of the gamble listeria presents, smoked fish—both hot (counting smoked mackerel and hot smoked salmon and pate) and cold (counting smoked salmon)—should now be avoided, except if they're completely cooked.

The Food Guidelines Office makes sense of:'Pregnancy-associated listeriosis can result in miscarriages as well as severe sepsis or meningitis in infants.

Dr. Caroline Handford, Acting Head of Occurrences at the Food Guidelines Organization, adds: "While the dangers to the overall population of turning out to be genuinely sick because of listeria are extremely low, we really want individuals who are helpless—specifically those older than 65, pregnant ladies, and individuals with debilitated safe frameworks—to know about the continuous dangers of consuming prepared-to-eat smoked fish. In the event that anybody from these gatherings is eating prepared-to-eat smoked fish, we are helping them to remember the exhortation to guarantee that it is entirely cooked before they eat it, including when filled in as a component of a dish.

"Meat ought to be cooked through totally because of the risk of toxoplasmosis-conveying parasites. This incorporates steaks, cooks, burgers, frankfurters, poultry, and pork.

Pepperoni, salami, chorizo, and air-dried hams might contain these parasites too, so the most secure choice is to eat them cooked.

- Liver, haggis, and pâté

In light of the great vitamin A substance, pregnant ladies are exhorted not to eat liver or items containing liver (wiener, pâté, and haggis). Pâté has an additional risk of listeria.

- Crude milk and crude yogurt

These food sources aren't broadly accessible, but they ought to be kept away from because of the risk of listeria defilement.

Supplements

- Folic corrosive

Pregnant ladies are encouraged to take a 400-microgram folic corrosive enhancement consistently all through the initial 12 weeks of their pregnancy. Folic corrosive assists with forestalling spinal imperfections (particularly spina bifida) as your child creates them. Food varieties, for example, salad greens, contain folic acid, and you ought to eat a lot of these, yet the levels you can get from diet alone aren't viewed as adequate enough for pregnant ladies.

- Vitamin D

All adults, including pregnant ladies, are urged to take a 10-microgram vitamin D supplement every day. Vitamin D is made by the body from openness to daylight, especially an issue in the colder time of year as well. Individuals who have a brown complexion or keep their skin very much covered outside presumably need to take an enhancement in the late spring as well.

- Iron

A few ladies experience the ill effects of iron deficiency during pregnancy. It's hard to tell whether exhaustion is brought about by this or by simply being pregnant. An eating regimen rich in red meat, nuts, and dried foods grown from ground greens might be sufficient to give you the iron you really want. Your PCP or maternity specialist will actually want to exhort in the event that you would profit from an enhancement too.

- Multivitamin supplements

There are multivitamin supplements targeted explicitly at pregnant women. Assuming you are attempting to eat due to queasiness or an ailment, these might be useful. High-portion multivitamins or any enhancements containing vitamin A ought to be kept away from. In the event that you're uncertain on the off chance that you really want a nutrient enhancement or which one to take, talk it over with your primary care physician or maternity specialist.

Conclusion

Dala B. Humphrey's pregnancy-friendly meal plan rises above the limits of traditional wholesome aides for eager moms. Through the fastidious embroidery she winds around, mixing clinical skill, compassion, and a festival of the groundbreaking idea of pregnancy, Humphrey makes an aide that is both useful and supportive.

As perusers venture through the pages, they experience functional dinner plans as well as witness a humane buddy in Humphrey. Her obligation to the all-encompassing prosperity of moms and unborn kids is obvious, making the pregnancy-friendly meal plan something other than a dietary guide—it turns into a demonstration of the significant magnificence and intricacy of the pre-birth insight.

Humphrey's work remains a reference point for hopeful moms, offering an abundance of information established in proof-based rehearsals while recognizing the profound and otherworldly components of pregnancy. The excursion delineated in this guide isn't just about nourishment; it's an investigation of taking care of oneself, satisfaction, and association, directed by the mastery and sympathy of the creator complexities of this exceptional section in a lady's life.

In the last pages of the pregnancy-friendly meal plan, perusers are left with an aide as well as a heritage—a tradition of shrewdness, empathy, and the resolute conviction that sustaining both body and soul is the way into an energetic and feeding pregnancy. Dala B. Humphrey welcomes each hopeful mother to embrace this excursion, advising them that the way to parenthood isn't just an actual undertaking but rather a significant festival of life, love, and the exceptional connection between mother and youngster.

.